Yoga for Fertility Handbook

By: Sue Dumais

Order this book online at www.trafford.com/08-1367
or email orders@trafford.com

Most Trafford titles are also available at major online book retailers.

Note for Librarians: A cataloguing record for this book is available from Library
and Archives Canada at www.collectionscanada.ca/amicus/index-e.html

Printed in Victoria, BC, Canada.

ISBN: 978-1-4251-8883-2

*We at Trafford believe that it is the responsibility of us all, as both individuals
and corporations, to make choices that are environmentally and socially sound.
You, in turn, are supporting this responsible conduct each time you purchase a
Trafford book, or make use of our publishing services. To find out how you are
helping, please visit www.trafford.com/responsiblepublishing.html*

*Our mission is to efficiently provide the world's finest, most comprehensive
book publishing service, enabling every author to experience success.
To find out how to publish your book, your way, and have it available
worldwide, visit us online at www.trafford.com/10510*

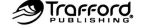

www.trafford.com

North America & international
toll-free: 1 888 232 4444 (USA & Canada)
phone: 250 383 6864 • fax: 250 383 6804
email: info@trafford.com

The United Kingdom & Europe
phone: +44 (0)1865 487 395 • local rate: 0845 230 9601
facsimile: +44 (0)1865 481 507 • email: info.uk@trafford.com

10 9 8 7 6 5 4 3 2 1

Acknowledgements

I would like to dedicate this book to all the women and couples struggling with fertility. I hope this book will inspire you and help you realize you are not alone. I want to thank everyone who has attended my Yoga for Fertility classes. I have learned so much from each of you, personally and professionally. It has truly been a gift. Together we have created a healing community that I know will continue to grow and expand, providing support all over the world.

I thank Dr. Wayne Dyer for his book Inspiration. His words and encouragement to follow my inner guidance inspired me to begin teaching my first Yoga for Fertility class.

Thank you to my sister-in-law Adrienne Thiessen of Gemini Visuals for all the beautiful photos. Thanks to Susanne Rutchinski for the beautiful design for my book cover. I thank my friend, my coach and soul sister Lisa Windsor. I am so grateful for your motivation and unwavering faith in me.

I thank my family for their patience and love. To my husband Steve who has encouraged me to follow my heart and surrounds me with unconditional love and support. I couldn't have asked for a better life partner to take this journey with.

I am so thankful for all the spirit babies and their willingness to communicate with me. You have touched my soul and I am honored to be of service to help you communicate with your parents.

I am grateful for my own inner guidance and courage to continue when times where tough. Although my fertility journey has been the most challenging time in my entire life, I deeply appreciate each and every experience. This has been such a rich and transforming journey. It has taught me to live fully, love without fear and trust in my Self.

Table of Contents

Introduction

Yoga for Fertility was conceived through my own personal struggle with fertility. The last 7 years have been an emotional roller coaster ride that affected every area of my life. My yoga practice continues to allow me to live through my fertility journey with trust and faith. When I began practicing Yoga for Fertility I discovered an incredible gift both physically and emotionally. I was able to release all the built up emotions and tension in my body from the years of stress and anxiety related to my fertility challenges. I no longer feel defeated and helpless. In fact I have never felt more in tune with my mind, body and soul as I do today. I have an inner strength and trust that walks with me, surrounding me and supporting me through every situation. I am at home in my heart and I hope that this book will help you find the deep sense of inner peace that I have found.

Yoga for Fertility

Yoga for fertility focuses on the centers of your body or "chakras" associated with fertility and reproduction. I have chosen specific poses that open your pelvis and stimulate your second chakra located just below your naval. This vital energy centre has long been associated with fertility and creativity. Releasing tension in your lower belly and pelvis will help increase the flow of blood and energy to your reproductive organs. Many of the poses in this book will also help reduce stress and anxiety and restore physical and emotional balance. Each pose offers an opportunity for you to create awareness. As you become aware you can begin to release physical tension, negative emotions and energetic blocks in the physical body that interfere with your fertility. Remember to begin where you are. No judgment. "I am where I am and it's ok".

Principles of Yoga for Fertility

I have created a list of the principles I believe capture the essence of Yoga for Fertility. In the blue column beside each yoga pose I have included some yoga principles that you can reflect on during that pose. I also encourage you to explore and reflect on each one of the principles by answering the questions below.

Breath	Acceptance
Trust	Awareness
Faith	Presence/Being
Hope	Grounded
Love	Centered
Forgiveness	Alignment
Self	Balance
Connection	Surrender

As you read each principle begin by choosing the one that speaks to you on a deep level. With your eyes closed, take a few breaths and repeat the word in your mind's eye or out loud if possible. Do this for at least 5 breaths then open your eyes and answer the following questions. Go with the first answers that come to your mind.

What does this principle mean to me?

How can I bring this principle into my yoga practice?

How can this principle help me in my fertility journey?

How can I bring this principle into my everyday life experiences?

Getting the Most out of your Practice

It is important that you listen to your body and the messages it gives you; before, during and after each pose. I encourage you to come into each pose at a level where you feel challenged by the pose and at the same time feel supported by your body or the props. There are many ways to modify the poses to increase comfort. There will be times that you may feel emotional. Be aware of how you are feeling. Accept and allow the emotion to be present. Listen deeply to your body and be guided by your own comfort. If something doesn't feel "right" then modify or dis-continue that pose. Notice that some poses will be challenging on more of an emotional or mental level. I encourage you to stay in these poses to explore them, remaining curious about all the lay-ers of your experience. As you listen to your inner guidance you will discover or remember, you are your best teacher.

Creating your Home Practice

You can use the program library on pages 35-38 for possible class combinations to begin your practice. As you become famil-iar with the different poses I encourage you to follow your own inner voice and guidance. When creating your own sequence choose a yoga pose that feels challenging - physically, mentally and emotionally. Also include a pose that speaks to you on a deep level, one that your body says "thank you" for doing. If you need further support I have created voice guided recordings of 60 minute classes to download on your computer, mp3 or iPod. Visit my website at www.familypassages.ca for more information.

Be sure to incorporate some meditation. See if you can sit qui-etly observing your body and mind for 5-10 minutes a day. Prac-tice mindfulness when you are eating or going for a walk. Yoga is not only something you practice on your mat; it is a way of living. To what extent can you bring your yoga practice into your life?

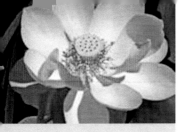

Mountain Pose

Stand tall in your body and feel connected to the earth.

Draw on your inner strength and personal power.

Feel your feet firmly planted in the earth.

Draw some of the nutrients from the earth and send negative energy into the earth like the roots of a tree.

This is a very grounding pose. As you root your feet deeply into the earth you can alert the mind and create balance – mind, body and spirit. Many clients feel out of control throughout their fertility journey and grounding can help you to connect to your inner guidance and receive the support and energy from the universe.

Preparation: Stand tall with feet close together (distance depends on individual comfort). Lift and spread your toes. Gently place your big toes on the floor first leaving your smaller toes up. Now slowly place your other toes down on the floor evenly spaced (do your best – in the beginning this is not easy for a lot of people). Press down into the floor with your big toes and feel a connection to your inner thigh muscles and deep core. Ensure the 4 corners of your feet are in contact with the floor (inner and outer area of the heel and ball of the foot).

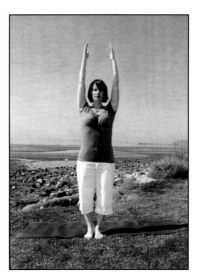

Modifications: Have a chair or wall close by if needed.

Option: Bring your arms above your head (as shown) and look toward the sky. Close your eyes to challenge your balance.

5

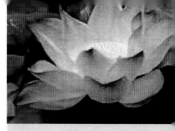

Extended Triangle Pose

This pose relieves stress and anxiety. It is a great pose for balance and it helps increase circulation to your pelvic area. This a great pose to help create space between your rib cage and pelvis by releasing tension in the waist. It is also known to improve function of your reproductive and digestive systems.

Preparation: Stand tall facing the front of your mat. Bring your left foot back and place it on the mat with a distance of about 3 feet between your feet. Turn your left foot on an angle with your left heel as the furthest point. Line your right heel with your left arch. Turn your torso to your left and raise your arms to shoulder height. Inhale and lift tall through your spine. Lift your left hip up slightly and as you exhale hinge at the hip bringing the right side of your torso and right arm/hand toward the floor and left arm/hand toward the sky. Take your gaze up, forward or down depending on your neck comfort. Keep your spine long and tall. Remember controlling the release is just as important as going into the pose. Repeat with the right foot back.

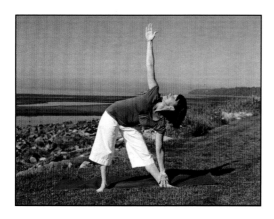

Modifications: Use a block or bolster under the hand closest to the floor for support.

Option: Close your eyes to challenge your balance.

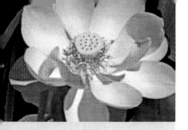

Centered

Imagine a balance between your two feet and then your fingertips. Now imagine this balance in your life.

Alignment

What would that feel like to have a sense of balance in my life?

Connection

Feel your body! Feel strong, alive and in control.

Warrior II

This pose focuses on stability, strength and balance. As you find a sense of balance in the pose, it can help you find a sense of balance in your life. This pose improves the effectiveness of your breath and overall circulation.

Preparation: Stand tall facing the front of your mat. Bring your left foot back and place it on the mat with a distance of about 3-4 feet from your right foot. Turn your left foot on an angle with your left heel as the furthest point. Line your right heel up with your left arch. Face your torso, pelvis and shoulders toward the left and raise your arms to the side up to shoulder height. Keep your shoulders above and in line with your pelvis. Find a way to balance the weight between your right and left foot as well as your right and left fingertips. Take your gaze forward looking beyond your fingertips.

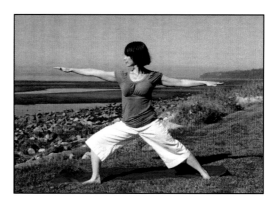

Modifications: Keep your feet closer together to help with balance.

Option: Close your eyes to challenge your balance.

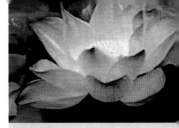

Tree Pose

This pose focuses on balance, stability and inner strength. It helps improve your concentration and focus.

Preparation: Stand tall with feet close together (distance depends on individual comfort). Lift and spread your toes. Gently place your big toes on the floor first leaving your smaller toes up. Slowly place your other toes down on the floor evenly spaced. Press down into the floor with your big toes and feel a connection to your inner thigh muscles and lower belly. Ensure contact with the floor with these 4 points (inner and outer area of your heel and ball of the foot). Place one heel on the inside of your opposite ankle with toes in contact with the floor, just above your knee or press your foot into your inner thigh. Choose a level where you feel supported yet challenged. Keep your eyes focused on something in front of you to help you with your balance.

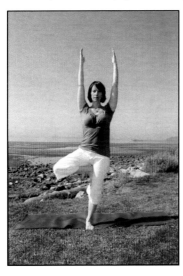

Modifications: Stand close to a wall or chair in case you need support.

Option: Place your hands in prayer at your heart center or extend your arms overhead to challenge your balance.

Balance

Imagine your foot reaching deep down into the earth and branching out like the roots of a tree.

Connection

Draw some of the nutrients from the earth and send negative energy down your roots.

Surrender

Imagine your worries falling like leaves from your branches. Simply letting go.

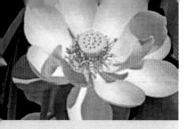

Awareness

Appreciate your body in the pose, make peace with the tension, and then invite softness.

Acceptance

Explore and embrace your resistance (physical or emotional).

Surrender

How can I surrender in this pose?

How can I surrender in my fertility journey?

Standing Forward Bend

This pose brings about a sense of peace and calm in your mind and body. It helps lift and tone your uterus and improves circulation to your pelvic area.

Preparation: Stand tall with feet close together (distance depends on individual comfort). Lift and spread the toes. Gently place your big toes on the floor first, leaving the smaller toes up. Now slowly place your other toes down on the floor evenly spaced (do your best – in the beginning this is not easy for a lot of people). Press down into the floor with your big toes and feel a connection to your inner thigh muscles and lower belly. Ensure the 4 corners of your feet are in contact with the floor (inner and outer area of the heel and ball of the foot). Reach your arms above your head inhaling to the sky. As you exhale hinge at your hips and allow your arms to float down toward the floor. Relax your sitz bones away from each other and let your head hang.

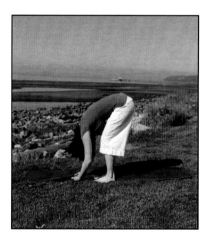

Modifications: Place your hands on a bolster in front of you or on your feet or legs if needed.

Option: Walk your hands side to side bringing your rib cage with you creating a stretch in your side body. It is important to leave your pelvis and sitz bones behind.

9

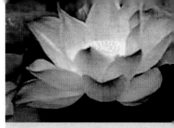

Wide Standing Forward Bend

This pose helps bring about a sense of peace and calm in your mind and body. It helps lift and tone your uterus and improves circulation to your pelvic area. It is also used to relieve heavy bleeding and to decrease the sense of heaviness during menstruation.

Preparation: Stand tall with your feet about 3 feet apart. Reach your arms above your head inhaling to the sky. As you exhale hinge at your hips and allow your arms to float down toward the floor. Relax your sitz bones away from each other and let your head hang.

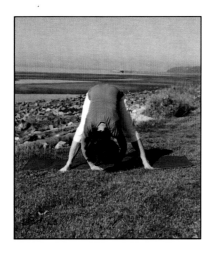

Modifications: Place your hands on a bolster or blocks in front of you.

Option: Use a chair in front of you for support to place your arms and hands.

Awareness

Appreciate your body in the pose, make peace with the tension, and then invite softness.

Acceptance

Explore and embrace your resistance (physical or emotional).

Surrender

How can I surrender in this pose?

How can I surrender in my fertility journey?

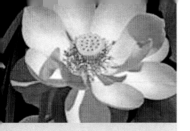

Appreciate your body in the pose, make peace with the tension, and then invite softness.

Acceptance

Explore and embrace your resistance (physical or emotional).

Surrender

How can I surrender in this pose?

How can I surrender in my fertility journey?

Seated Forward Bend

This pose relieves anxiety by creating a sense of calm in your mind. It also helps stimulate your ovaries and uterus.

Preparation: Sit tall on the sitz bones of your pelvis. Reach your arms above your head inhaling to the sky as you lengthen through your spine. As you exhale, hinge at your hips and allow your arms to float down toward your legs. Relax your sitz bones away from each other and let your head hang. Invite softness from your tailbone toward your upper spine melting tension as you bring your awareness up your spine.

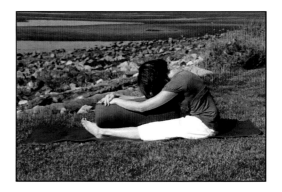

Modifications: Place your butt cheeks on a yoga block while keeping your sitz bones in contact with the floor. This may provide support for your pelvis and lower back and assist you in keeping your spine tall.

Option: Place a bolster or pillow on your lap to support your arms and head (as shown).

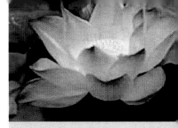

Wide-Angle Seated Pose

This pose will help increase circulation to your pelvis. It helps regulate your menstrual flow and stimulate your ovaries.

Preparation: Sit tall on the sitz bones of the pelvis. Move your legs away from each other until you feel a mild to moderate stretch in your inner thigh muscles. Place your hands on the floor in front of you or behind to provide support to help you remain tall through the spine.

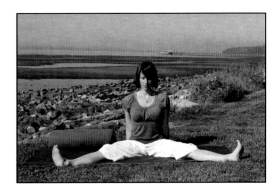

Modifications: Place your butt cheeks on a yoga block while keeping your sitz bones in contact with the floor. This may provide support for your pelvis and lower back and assist you in keeping your spine tall as well as keeping your pelvic floor parallel to the ground.

Option: Perform this pose with your back against the wall for support.

Grounded

Imagine your pelvis was the trunk of a tree with roots deep into the earth.

Connection & Centered

Connect to your inner strength and wisdom. Feel tall through the spine and connect to the universe through your crown.

Faith

I am exactly where I need to be.

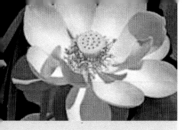

Awareness

Appreciate
your body in
the pose,
make peace
with the
tension, and
then invite
softness.

Acceptance

Explore and
embrace your
resistance
(physical or
emotional).

Surrender

How can I
surrender in
this pose?

How can I
surrender in
my fertility
journey?

Wide-Angle Seated Pose with Twist

This pose will help increase circulation to your pelvic area, regulate menstrual flow and stimulate your ovaries and kidneys.

Preparation: Sit tall on the sitz bones of your pelvis. Move your legs away from each other until you feel a mild to moderate stretch in your inner thigh muscles. Inhale and lengthen through your spine, exhale as you twist through your waist toward your left leg. Fold your upper body and allow yourself to relax toward your left leg. Place your hands on your leg or floor and let your head hang. Repeat on the right.

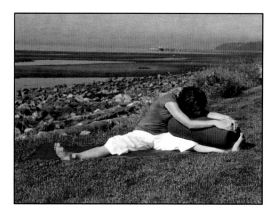

Modifications: Place your butt cheeks on a yoga block while keeping your sitz bones in contact with the floor. This may provide support for your pelvis and lower back and assist you in keeping your spine tall.

Option: Place a bolster or pillow on your lap to support your arms and head (as shown).

13

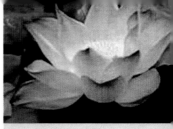

Wide-Angle Seated Forward Bend

This pose can improve blood circulation in your pelvic area and help regulate your menstrual flow. This pose has a calming effect that can help reduce irritability.

Preparation: Sit tall on the sitz bones of the pelvis. Move your legs away from each other until you feel a mild to moderate stretch in your inner thigh muscles. Reach your arms above your head inhaling to the sky as you lengthen through your spine. As you exhale, hinge at your hips and allow your arms to float down toward the floor. Relax your sitz bones away from each other and let your head hang. Invite softness from your tailbone toward your upper spine melting tension as you bring your awareness up your spine.

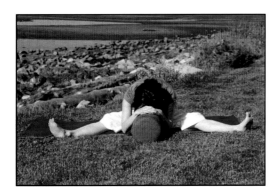

Modifications: Place your butt cheeks on a yoga block while keeping your sitz bones in contact with the floor. This may provide support for your pelvis and lower back and assist you in keeping your spine tall.

Option: Place a bolster or pillow between your legs to support or rest your arms and head (as shown).

Awareness

Appreciate your body in the pose, make peace with the tension, and then invite softness.

Acceptance

Explore and embrace your resistance (physical or emotional).

Surrender

How can I surrender in this pose?

How can I surrender in my fertility journey?

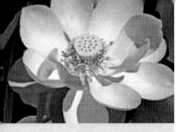

Alignment

As you inhale invite your spine to lengthen, as you exhale invite softness in your muscles and melt tension.

Acceptance

Explore and embrace your resistance (physical or emotional). "I am where I am and it's ok"

Trust

Trust in the wisdom of your body. Listen to the messages it sends you.

Simple Seated Twist

This pose provides a gentle twist to massage your reproductive organs. It helps to energize your adrenal glands and tone your kidneys. The gentleness of this twist is safe at any time in the menstrual cycle including early pregnancy. Be guided by your own comfort.

Preparation: Bend your knees and swing the lower part of your legs to the right, resting your knees and feet on the floor. As you inhale, lift tall through your spine and as you exhale, twist through your waist toward the left. Take your head and your gaze toward the left.

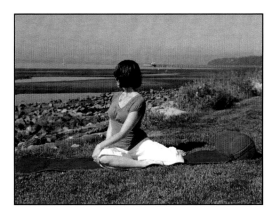

Modifications: Use a block under the hand behind the back to provide more support for the spine and to cushion the wrist if needed.

Option: Sit with legs crossed.

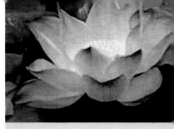

Head on Knee Pose

This cooling pose has a toning effect on your reproductive organs. It can be beneficial for relieving menstrual cramps and symptoms of PMS. It is a great pose to help reduce anxiety.

Preparation: Sit tall on the sitz bones of the pelvis with one leg straight out in front of you and tuck your other leg in with your knee bent. Reach your arms above your head inhaling to the sky as you lengthen through your spine. As you exhale, hinge at your hips and allow your arms to float down toward your straight leg. Relax your sitz bones away from each other and let your head hang. Invite softness from your tailbone toward your upper spine melting tension as you bring your awareness up your spine. Repeat using the other leg.

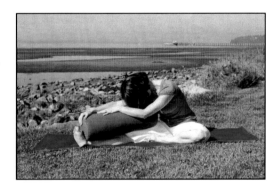

Modifications: Place your butt cheeks on a yoga block while keeping your sitz bones in contact with the floor. This may provide support for your pelvis and lower back and assist you in keeping your spine tall.

Option: Place a bolster or pillow on your leg to support or rest your arms and head (as shown).

Awareness

Appreciate your body in the pose, make peace with the tension, and then invite softness.

Acceptance

Explore and embrace your resistance (physical or emotional).

Surrender

How can I surrender in this pose?

How can I surrender in my fertility journey?

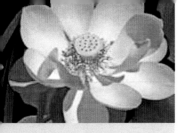

Cat Pose

This pose is a great stretch for your entire back and spine. It helps bring your awareness to the present moment and warm up the spine as you link the movement with your breath.

Preparation: Start in a 4 point kneeling position with your hands under your shoulders and knees directly under your hips. Inhale as you prepare. As you exhale begin to arch and round your back, tucking your tailbone under and bringing your head down looking toward your knees. Continue to breathe as you hold this position.

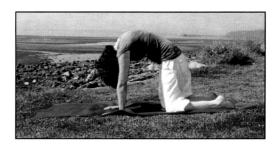

Modifications: Place a bolster, blankets or blocks under your wrists for cushioning.

Option: Link with Cow Pose and flow with your breath. Inhaling as you move into Cow Pose and exhale as you move into Cat Pose. Close your eyes and be guided by your breath.

Breath

Link your movement with breath to experience meditation in movement.

Presence/ Being

What is it like to be with SELF? What is happening right now?

Self

As you look inward, to what extent can you appreciate your mind and body?

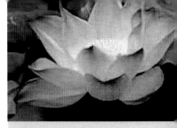

Cow Pose

This is a great pose to warm up the back and spine. It helps bring awareness to the present moment as you link the movement with your breath.

Preparation: Start in a 4 point kneeling position with your hands under your shoulders and knees directly under your hips. Exhale as you prepare. As you inhale begin to move your belly toward the floor, lifting your head and tailbone. Continue to breathe as you hold this position.

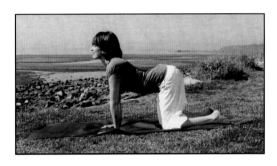

Modifications: Place a bolster, blankets or blocks under your wrists for cushioning.

Option: Link with Cat Pose and flow with your breathe. Inhaling as you move into Cow Pose and exhale as you move into Cat Pose. Close your eyes and be guided by your breath.

Awareness

Be curious about any sensations, emotions, images, memories or thoughts you experience. No judgment, just be aware.

Breath

Link your movement with breath to experience meditation in movement.

Love

As I lift my head and open my heart to life. I open my heart to love.

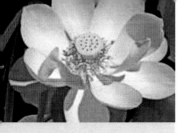

Presence/
Being

Be aware of
the physical,
mental and
emotional
body.
Appreciate
how your body
is supporting
you.

Hope

Focus on your
desire to have
a baby. Invite
an openness to
conceive and
an openness to
life.

Self

Find strength
in
vulnerability.

Bridge Pose

This is an energizing pose. It helps tone your kidneys and adrenal glands. It is also known to help regulate your menstrual cycle. It is great for strengthening your uterus and ovaries.

Preparation: Lay on your back with your knees bent and feet on the floor. Start with a neutral spine. Place your hands by your sides pressing your triceps into the floor. Slowly lift your sacrum and pelvis off the floor while pressing your lower back flat in to the floor. As you lift your hips roll your shoulders underneath you and place the weight across the back of your shoulders while pressing your hands and triceps in to the floor. Keep your knees in line with the hip joints. I do not recommend this pose during menstruation.

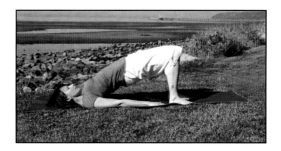

Modifications: Place a bolster, blankets or blocks under your pelvis/sacrum for a supported bridge.

Option: Use a strap to wrap around the thighs to keep your knees in line with your hips.

19

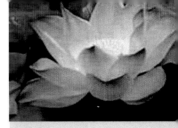

Seated Bound Angle Pose

This pose strengthens your bladder and uterus. It also helps tone your kidneys. It can help ease symptoms of PMS, menstrual cramps and heavy bleeding.

Preparation: Sit tall on the sitz bones of the pelvis. Wrap and secure the strap around your pelvis and ankles as shown in the photo below.

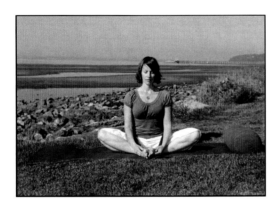

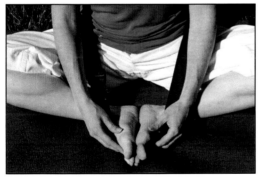

Modifications: Place your butt cheeks on a yoga block while keeping your sitz bones in contact with the floor. This may provide support for the pelvis and lower back and assist you in keeping your spine tall as well as keeping your pelvic floor parallel to the ground.

Option: Perform this pose without the strap. Sit with your back against the wall for support.

Imagine your pelvis was the trunk of a tree with roots deep into the earth.

Connection& Centered

Connect to your inner strength and wisdom. Feel tall through the spine and connected to the universe through your crown.

Faith

I am exactly where I need to be.

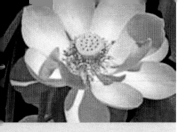

Reclined Bound Angle Pose

This pose is designed to open the front of your body and your pelvis. It also provides a deep stretch for your lower back. It helps take pressure off your pelvic area, relieves menstrual cramps, heaviness or spasms in the uterus. With the arms resting to the side, you will experience an opening of your chest and 4th chakra (giving and receiving love). It is great to help clear your mind and calm your nerves.

Preparation: Place a bolster or blankets behind you right up against the back of your pelvis. Wrap and secure the strap around your pelvis and ankles as shown in the photo. The length of the strap should be determined by your comfort level once you lie back. Slowly lower your back onto the bolster. Release your arms out to the side with your palms facing up to open your chest.

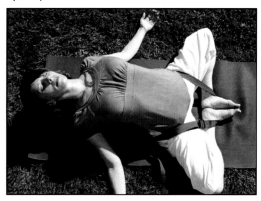

Modifications: This pose is ideally performed using a bolster under your back. The higher the bolster, the more intense the stretch. Choose a height that feels comfortable on your back and pelvis. Use blankets or blocks instead of a bolster to adjust the height.

Option: This pose can be done without the strap. To come out of the pose gently place your elbows and hands on the floor beside you and slowly push yourself up.

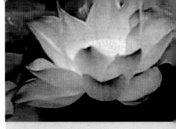

Child's Pose

This pose calms your nervous system, helps reduce blood pressure and balances the endocrine system. It is a resting pose that relaxes and calms your mind and body while lengthening your spine and reducing tension in your back and neck. In relation to fertility, I recommend performing child's pose with your knees apart; this allows space for your belly to drop toward the floor with each inhale. Imagine softness in your uterus and ovaries allowing the flow of blood and energy without restriction or tension.

Preparation: Kneel on the floor with your knees slightly wider than your hip joints. Keep your feet together. Sit back with your hips and bring your chest toward the floor. Reach your arms forward and place your hands and forehead on the floor.

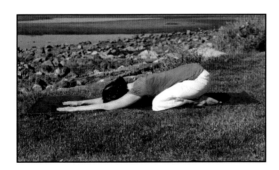

Modifications: If there is a space between your heels and pelvis place a block to provide support. You can use a bolster or pillow under your head and arms or bend your elbows and place your hands under your forehead.

Option: Turtle Pose - Place your hands beside your feet or ankles creating more security and safety as you settle into your "shell" for protection.

Self

Reflect on your relationship with SELF. Do I speak kindly to myself? Am I my own best friend?

Forgiveness

Is there anyone or anything I need to forgive?

Love

Do you love yourself? Reflect on a time as a child when you adored yourself.

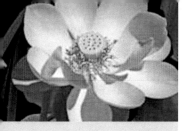

Awareness

Notice any
tension in the
lower belly
and pelvis?

Connection

Invite soft-
ness and space
in your lower
belly and pel-
vis. Imagine a
beautiful,
warm and
nourishing
space in your
uterus for
your baby.

Love

Surround your
reproductive
organs with
love and
healing
energy.

Legs-Up-The-Wall Pose

This pose will increase the blood supply to your pelvic area, calm the mind and relieve tired legs and feet. If you focus on expanding your belly with each inhale, it will help you soften the muscles of your vaginal wall and pelvic area. Imagine softness in your uterus and ovaries allowing the flow of blood and energy without restriction or tension.

Preparation: Lie on your side with your buttocks close to or against the wall. As you slowly roll over onto your back gently lift one leg at a time and place it against the wall. Once you are on your back, rest the legs against the wall. Stay in this pose for 5-15 minutes as you concentrate on your breathing. To come out of the pose gently bend your knees and roll over on to your side remaining on your side for 10 to 15 breaths.

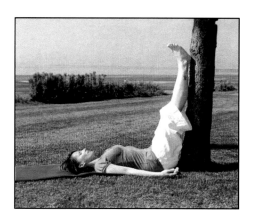

Modifications: This pose can be performed using a bolster, block or blanket under the pelvis. The blanket or bolster should lift the pelvis approximately 2-3 inches depending on your level of comfort. *DO NOT use a bolster with this pose during menstruation.

Option: Move your legs away from each other creating a mild stretch for your inner thigh.

23

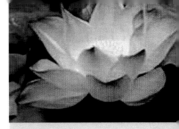

Side Body Stretch

This pose will help improve your breath through the sides of your body by creating space and softness in the muscles of your waist. Melting tension in your back and side body can improve your breath and increase the amount of oxygen you inhale into your lungs, resulting in more oxygen circulating in your blood stream.

Preparation: Sit tall in a crossed legged position. Reach your right arm up while keeping your right shoulder relaxed down. As you exhale lean your body over to the left bringing your right ribs along and leaving the right hip behind. Invite the ribs on the right to expand with each inhale and softly return with each exhale. Stay in this pose for at least 10-20 breaths. Pause in the center to compare right and left side before repeating with your left arm.

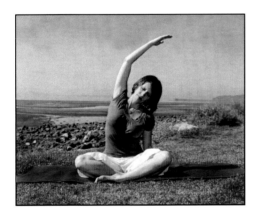

Modifications: Place a bolster on your left side to provide support for your left arm.

Option: Place your hand on your right rib cage to feel the expansion with each inhale.

Awareness

Appreciate your body in the pose, make peace with the tension, and then invite softness.

Breath

Become your breath. Invite a longer exhale creating space for a longer inhale. Encourage your breath to reach deeper into your lungs.

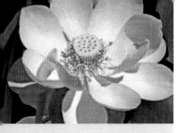

Awareness

Appreciate
your body,
make peace
with the
tension and
then invite
softness.

Acceptance

Explore and
embrace any
anger or
frustration.
Make peace
with where
you are.

Forgiveness

Who do I
need to
forgive?
Do I need to
forgive
myself?

Pigeon

This pose will help create space in your pelvis and hips. The hips are a common place to hold anger and frustration which will often show up in the physical body as tension. Releasing this blocked energy can help increase blood and circulation to your hips, pelvis and reproductive organs.

Preparation: From a four point kneeling position, bring your right leg forward and hook it in front of your left knee. Keeping your right knee bent, slide your left leg back straightening your left leg to the floor. Keep your hips level by using props on either side of your pelvis. Encourage a slight internal rotation of the left thigh, knee and foot. Hold this pose for 2-5 minutes. Repeat with your left leg forward.

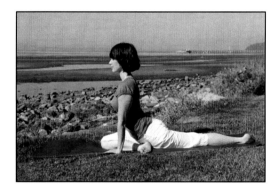

Modifications: Place your butt cheek on a blanket or yoga block.

Option: Walk your arms forward and relax your upper body toward the floor.

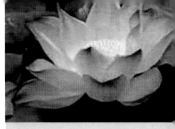

Hip/Glute Stretch

This pose will help create space in your pelvis and hips. The hips are a common place to hold anger and frustration which will often show up in the physical body as tension. Releasing this blocked energy can help increase blood and circulation to your hips, pelvis and reproductive organs.

Preparation: Lay on your back with your knees bent. Place your right ankle onto the left lower thigh. Bring both legs in toward your chest and hold the left leg with your hands. Encourage the right knee to rotate out away from your chest.

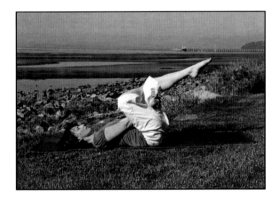

Modifications: Use a strap wrapped around your left thigh instead of your hands. This will allow you to rest your head and neck on the floor and prevent any unnecessary tension in your upper body.

Option: Perform this pose in a seated position on a chair.

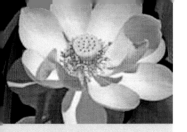

Notice the physical body before and after the exercise. How do I feel before the exercise? Where am I holding negative energy or emotion?

Presence/ Being

What is happening now? Be with yourself and be guided by your own inner wisdom. How can I invite a sense of calm and inner peace?

Shake it off!

This is a very playful way to release or shift any stuck energy from your physical body. Like water off a duck's back this exercise allows you to let go without attachment. Just let it roll off. Anytime you feel frustrated or irritated by something, try this exercise. I promise you will be pleasantly surprised at how effective and easy it is to let go.

Preparation: Lay on your back with your arms and legs in the air. Shake your arms and legs in whatever way feels good. Be guided by your own comfort and move whatever way you want. Shake for about 10-30 seconds then release your arms and legs to the floor. Be aware of the physical sensations. Notice your arms, hands, fingers, legs, feet and toes. Be aware of your emotions. Do you still feel the negative emotion or have your shaken it loose? Repeat as needed.

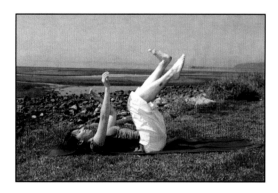

Modifications: Start with shaking the arms only or legs only.

Option: Shake it off while standing. There are no rules! Just do what feels good.

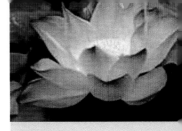

Corpse Pose

This pose is a great way to end your yoga practice. It is relaxing and soothing and helps reduce anxiety. It is helpful to restore balance. This pose is extremely important in integrating all the benefits of your yoga session. Resist the temptation to skip it. Give yourself permission to "do nothing" and notice your body and mind in stillness.

Preparation: Lay on your back on a comfortable surface, close your eyes and breathe.

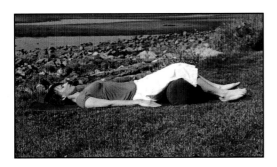

Modifications: Place a bolster under your knees to provide support for the pelvis and lower back (as shown).

Option: Place a blanket over you and an eye pillow.

Being/ Presence

Give yourself permission to find stillness. Notice how you feel in mind, body and spirit.

Alignment

"I will align myself with my inner guidance. I will listen to the voice of my soul".

Love

Fill your body and soul with love and gratitude.

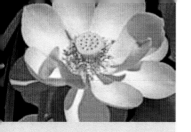

Meditation

Here are some mini meditations you can incorporate into your practice. Try them all and choose the one that works best for you. It is very normal for your thoughts to wander, gently bring your focus back to the meditation. As you practice, it will become easier. To complete, bring your awareness back to your body and your physical surroundings before opening your eyes.

Observing the Mind

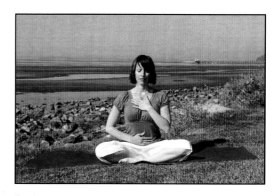

Close your eyes and bring your awareness to your breath for 5 breaths. Move your awareness to your mind. Begin to observe your thoughts. No judgment, just observe. Notice how your thoughts come and go. Observe the speed of your thoughts. Are they positive or negative? Imagine a balloon or bubble surrounding each thought and watch each thought float away. Begin to slow the thoughts by imagining you are slowing the speed. Notice whether there are spaces between the thoughts. Begin to invite positive and supportive thoughts such as "I believe" "I am strong" "I am fertile". Notice how the physical body changes as you begin to invite these new thoughts.

Presence/
Being

Notice what is happening in the mind. No judgment, no need to change anything, just observe.

Acceptance

"I am where I am and I am ok".

"I love my body and trust its' wisdom".

Faith

"I am strong"
"I am fertile"
"I believe"

29

Meditation

Breathing Meditations

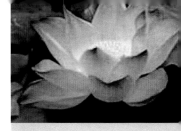

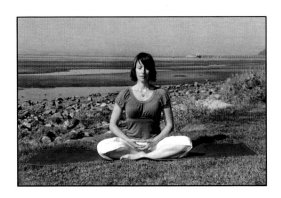

Breath

"I am grateful for my breath and the rhythm it creates. The more I stop and listen, the less I sit and wait".

Presence/ Being

Notice what is happening with your breath. No judgment, no need to change any- thing. Just observe.

A. Breath Awareness: Close your eyes and bring your aware- ness to your breath. Without changing the breath, notice the length of each inhale and each exhale. Notice how the exhale naturally follows each inhale. Become aware of the areas where the breath flows easily. Notice the areas where the breath has more of a challenge reaching. Remember there is no judgment, just observation. Is there a pause between the inhale and exhale or does one flow directly into the other? Listen, feel and allow the breath.

B. Counting the Breath: Close your eyes and bring your awareness to your breath. Begin to count for the length with each inhale (1, 2, 3, 4) and count the length of each exhale (1, 2, 3, 4, 5). Is the inhale longer or the same length as the exhale? Again there is no judgment just observe. Continue to count each breath in and out for 5-10 minutes.

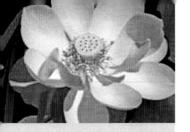

Presence/ Being

Notice what is happening in the mind. No judgment, no need to change anything, just observe.

Acceptance

"I am where I am and I am ok".

"I love my body and trust its' wisdom".

Faith

"I am strong"
"I am fertile"
"I believe"

Meditation

Affirmation Meditation

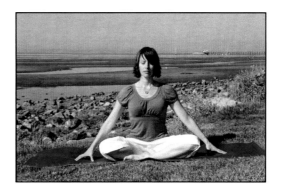

Close your eyes and bring your awareness to the breath. Reflect for a moment and ask yourself what you need for support in this moment. Allow the word to come intuitively from within. As you inhale repeat the words "I am" and on the exhale repeat the word you chose such as "calm" or "relaxed" or "trust". Invite the word into your body and create a felt sense of it. Repeat for 10-20 breaths or until you reach the desired effect.

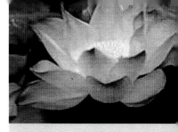

Meditation

Mindful Meditation

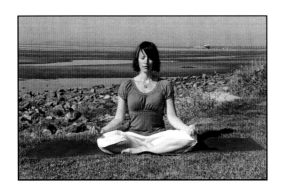

Practicing mindfulness while you are eating or walking allows you to become present. Being in the moment will help you focus your thoughts on the "now" versus an upcoming appointment or the 2 week wait for a pregnancy test. Practicing present moment awareness will keep you focused on "what is" and you will learn to shift your thoughts away from worrying about what may or may not happen in the future.

Initially, the process of re-training your mind and regaining control of your thoughts can be frustrating. I suggest you start with 5 minutes a day. It will get easier each time you meditate. There will be days where your thoughts are harder to slow. You may want to repeat in your mind or out loud "I am where I am and it is ok" and/or "My mind is busy and it is ok". As you move from judgment to acceptance, you will feel a sense of control and calm. Be patient!

Awareness

Bring your awareness to your senses. Focus on what you see, smell, hear, taste and feel.

Self

What have I learned about my SELF in my fertility journey? What am I grateful for?

Acceptance

I am exactly where I need to be.

How to Communicate with your Spirit Baby

After my miscarriage I was completely devastated. I was angry with myself, with the universe and anyone else I could blame for taking my baby away from me. I desperately wanted my baby to come back to me. I felt a deep sense of loss that grew heavier as each month passed. I kept asking "Why won't she come back to me?" One day a friend answered "Maybe the baby needs more time." Suddenly I realized it was not just about me and my husband, it was about the baby as well.

This sparked a deep sense of knowing there was much more to my fertility than just getting pregnant. When I first picked up the book "Spirit Babies" by Walter Makichen I couldn't put it down. I read the entire book in a couple of days. I was fascinated by the idea that my spirit baby will choose me as his/her mother. I was also comforted and empowered by the thought that I chose my parents as well.

Even in spirit our babies have different personalities with different needs. Your spirit baby can be around you for years before they decide to come into physical form, even long before you made the decision to have a child. Some babies need some encouragement, some are afraid, and others need to know that you and your partner are truly ready to have them in your life.

While in the yoga poses take some time to connect to your baby to be. Legs-Up-The-Wall Pose or Reclining Bound Angle Pose are great postures to use for this exercise. Here are some of the ways you can invite your baby to communicate with you.

Find stillness and bring your awareness to your breath (for at least 15-20 breaths). Repeat the following sentence out loud if possible. "Dear Spirit Baby, I invite you in on an energetic level so I can feel you in this reality." Be open and curious about any change in temperature, a sense of presence, an image, color or thought that comes to you. If you don't feel anything that doesn't mean your baby is not around you. Your spirit baby will often have a certain way of communicating with you. As you lower your resistance and become more open you may be able to hear words or see images. One of my spirit babies would hold my right hand and I would feel a warmth and pressure in my palm. The little spirit baby that is currently around me will softly place her hand on my right cheek when I invite her in to communicate with me. Once you invite them in, speak to them using words that come from your heart. Begin to mother them.

Here are some examples of what you can say until you find your own words. "I love you and I am ready for you to come into my life." "I am ready for you. You are safe. I will take care of you." You might even ask "Is there anything you need from me (us)?" Then clear space in your mind's eye for a message.

Many of the Spirit Babies are eager to communicate and I recommend you begin using your yoga practice to open the door of communication. If you need further guidance I offer private consultations and facilitate workshops to help strengthen your relationship with your baby to be. Visit www.familypassages.ca for more information.

Practicing Gratitude

Practicing gratitude allows you to shift your attention from what isn't working in your life to what is. Start with something unrelated to your fertility. Be grateful for the moon, nature, a delicious meal or the comfort of your pet. Really create a felt sense of gratitude in your heart and experience how your energy shifts. At the end of each day find 3 things you are grateful for and write them down. Take a moment to reflect on your fertility journey. Find one thing that you are grateful for. Perhaps the support of your partner or family. Maybe something you discovered about yourself. Observe how feeling gratitude can fill you up with hope and possibility.

Possible Class Combinations:

Here are some class combinations that you can follow for your own practice. Be sure to follow your inner guidance. I encourage you to begin each session with a meditation. Use which ever meditation speaks to you that day.

Class Combination #1 (Awareness & Acceptance)

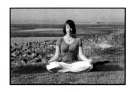

1. Meditation

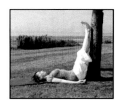

2. Legs-Up-The-Wall

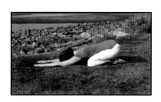

3. Child's pose

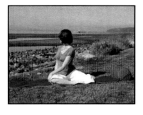

4. Seated twist

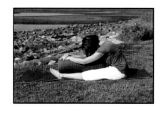

5. Seated forward bend

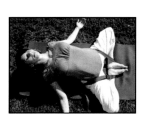

6. Reclined bound angle

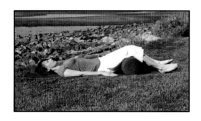

7. Corpse pose

Class Combination #2 (Forgiveness & Surrender)

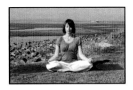

1. Meditation

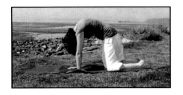

2. Cat/Cow Combination with Breath

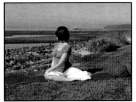 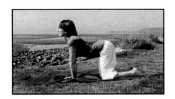

3. Seated twist   4. Wide angle seated pose with a twist

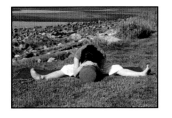 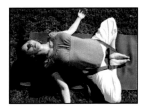

5. Wide forward bend   6. Reclined bound angle

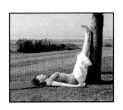 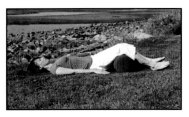

7. Legs-Up-The-Wall   8. Corpse pose

Class Combination #3 (Grounding & Connection)

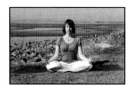

1. Meditation

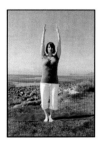

2. Mountain pose

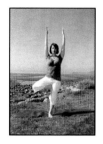

3. Tree pose

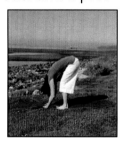

4. Standing forward bend

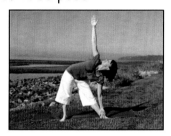

5. Triangle

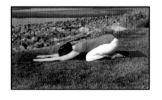

6. Child's pose

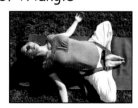

7. Reclined bound angle

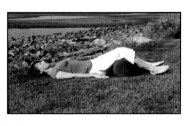

8. Corpse pose

Class Combination #4 (Love & Trust)

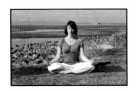

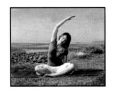

1. Meditation

2. Side body stretch

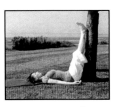

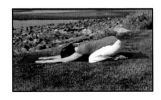

3. Legs-Up-The-Wall

4. Child's pose (reaching side to side)

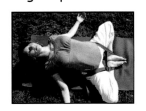

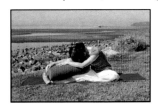

5. Reclined bound angle

6. Head on knee pose

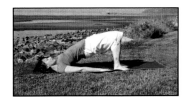

7. Bridge pose

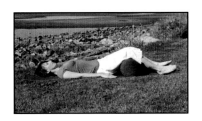

8. Corpse pose

Self Reflection

One day after your meditation or yoga practice I encourage you to answer the following questions. Use the next page or write your thoughts in your journal. These questions are meant to create awareness. Be curious. Be open. No judgment.

1. Take a moment to reflect on your fertility journey. What are the first words/thoughts that come to mind?
2. What words do I use to describe my body?
3. What words come to mind when I think about my uterus, ovaries and fallopian tubes?
4. Un-forgiveness is a toxin in your body. Who or what do I need to forgive?
5. What have I learned about myself throughout my fertility journey?
6. To what extent can I make peace with my past?

When it comes to shifting your perspective Awareness is the first key. The moment you become aware change has already begun.

The second step is Acceptance. It is important to make peace with where you are. "I am where I am and it's ok" "I am angry and it's ok" Remember acceptance doesn't mean you want to stay where you are.

The final step is Action. What is one thing you can do to help you move from where you are? Keep in mind sometimes the Action step is no action or the action is in the acceptance of what is.

An easy way to remember these steps is the 3 A's.
Awareness, Acceptance and Action.

Personal Notes:

Conclusion

I have created this handbook as a resource to help transform your fertility journey. Remember the most important teacher, is the one within yourself. Follow your inner guidance and listen to the wisdom and messages from your body and experience a rich and transforming yoga practice.

Begin to bring your yoga practice into ever day life situations. Follow your heart and it will lead you down the path toward your dream.

Believe, have faith and trust in your SELF!

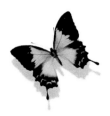

Anything is Possible

By: Sue Dumais

As you learn to follow your heart
You are guided by your inner wisdom

As you learn to believe in your dream
You remain in a place of hope

As you connect to your sense of Self
You find a place called home

When you are at home in your heart
You can move mountains

As you embrace your power within
Anything is possible

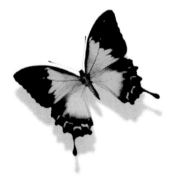

About the Author

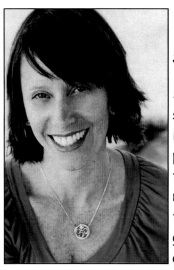

Sue Dumais

Sue Dumais is the founder of Family Passages Mind Body Studio in Vancouver, British Columbia, where she facilitates programs to support women and couples through their fertility. Sue combines more than 15 years of experience as a fitness expert, yoga instructor, energetic healer and life coach. She is the author of "A Strong Core for Life," and "Yoga for Fertility Handbook." She travels across Canada and internationally to teach and lecture on the importance of healing through one's fertility journey. Recognizing the need for more support for fertility clients, Sue has developed a Fitness Fertility Specialist Certification and Yoga for Fertility Instructor Training Course. A pioneer in her field, Sue's Yoga for Fertility Classes, Private Yoga Therapy Sessions and "Transforming Your Fertility" Teleclasses have been instrumental in transforming the fertility experiences of countless women and couples.

Resources

A STRONG CORE FOR LIFE, A Guide to Finding Your Deep Core Muscles. By Sue Dumais. Published by Trafford Publishing (2007)

INSPIRATION, Your Ultimate Calling. By Dr. Wayne Dyer. Published by Hay House Inc (2006)

TAKING CHARGE OF YOUR FERTILITY, The Definitive Guide to Natural Birth Control, Pregnancy Achievement and Reproductive Health. By Toni Weschler, MPH. Published by HarperCollins Publisher Inc (2002)

SPIRIT BABIES, How to Communicate with the Child You're Meant to Have. By Walter Makichen. Published by Bantam Dell (2005)

THE FEMALE PELVIS – Anatomy and Exercises. By Calais-Germain B. Published by Eastland Press Inc (2003)

THE INFERTILITY CURE, The Ancient Chinese Wellness Program for Getting Pregnant and Having Healthy Babies. By Randine Lewis PhD. Published by Little, Brown and Company (2004)

THE WAY OF THE FERTILE SOUL, Ten Ancient Chinese Secrets to Tap into a Women's Creative Potential. By Randine Lewis. Published by Beyond Words Publishing (2007)

YOGA FOR WOMEN. By Shakta Kaur Khalsa, Published by DK Publishing (2002)

THE FORGOTTEN BODY, A Way of Knowing and Understanding Self. By Elissa Cobb. Published by Satya House Publications (2008)

HEALING MIND, HEALTHY WOMEN, using the Mind Body Connection to manage stress and take control of your life. By Alice D Domar PhD and Henry Dreher. Published by Delta trade Paperbacks (1996)

ISBN 142518883-4